Unreported Truths about COVID-19, Cataclysms & World Lockdowns:

2020-2021 All Info You Need to Know about Covid-19, Coronavirus Conspiracy Theories, Outbreak, Education After Virus and Much More!

ISBN: : 9798584815660

CONTENTS

Introduction

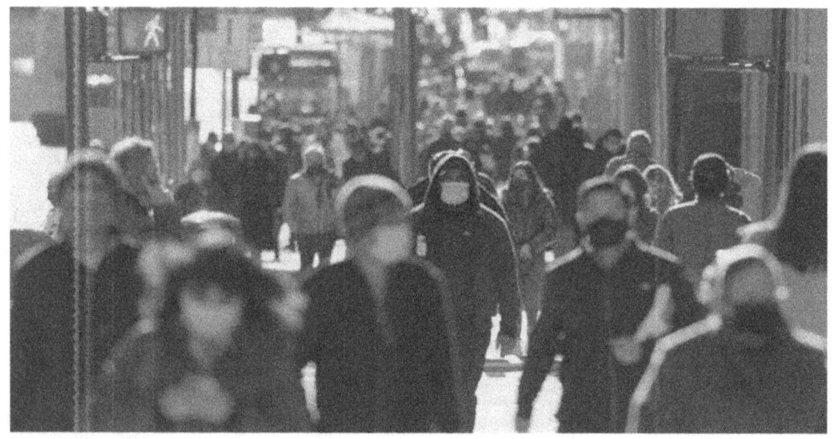

Talking about COVID-19, there is an uncontrollable amount of misinformation circulating on the internet. The sad part is that the wrong information easily misleads people. Even though the internet has more authentic information than misleading information, people still go for the latter. This is why it's important to know the types of coronaviruses, conspiracies, and other related information that you are likely to get confused with.

There could be many problems in believing misinformation; one of the recent events that happened in Sri Lanka was related to fish markets. During the second wave, almost all the COVID-19 positive cases were from the fish markets, so people panicked and stopped buying fish. This led to a massive fall in the fisheries industry, and daily wage earners were down with no income. Thus, the fisheries industry's ex-minister bit into raw fish to show that the people will not be contaminated by eating fish. The ex-minister's weird act circulated and received a lot of criticism from Sri Lankan Twitter, but after a week, the fisheries industry saw a spike in sales because of his act. Likewise, there have been a lot of consequences because of misinformation.

Although coronavirus is a new term for most of us, it is actually not. Coronaviruses have been in the world. There are different types of coronaviruses, but people weren't aware of it before COVID-19 came into the picture. Only after this pandemic people have actually made an effort to understand more about the types of viruses.

To understand about coronaviruses, you need to know what exactly it is. It is a family of viruses that create illness in animals and humans. There are different types of viruses found in humans; they are the viruses responsible for pandemics, including MERS, SARS, and COVID-19. Every report discusses the contagiousness of the virus and how every new virus is deadlier than another.

However, the world has changed a lot since the coronavirus came into the world, and people started to adapt to the new normal. There are several things that we need to learn and educate ourselves on. For example, the way people studied before the pandemic was totally different from the way they studying now. It has become nearly impossible to run a day without an internet connection. We must have a proper understanding of online teaching, online learning, online business, etc. Until an effective vaccine is found, we'll continue to live with the new normal lifestyle.

Here are some of the things that we'll discuss in this eBook, and I hope you will find them useful:

- Coronaviruses
- COVID-19 conspiracy theories
- The Future After COVID-19
- Education of the Future

These are some of the integral sections that we must know about the coronaviruses, so let's get started!

Chapter 1 – Coronaviruses

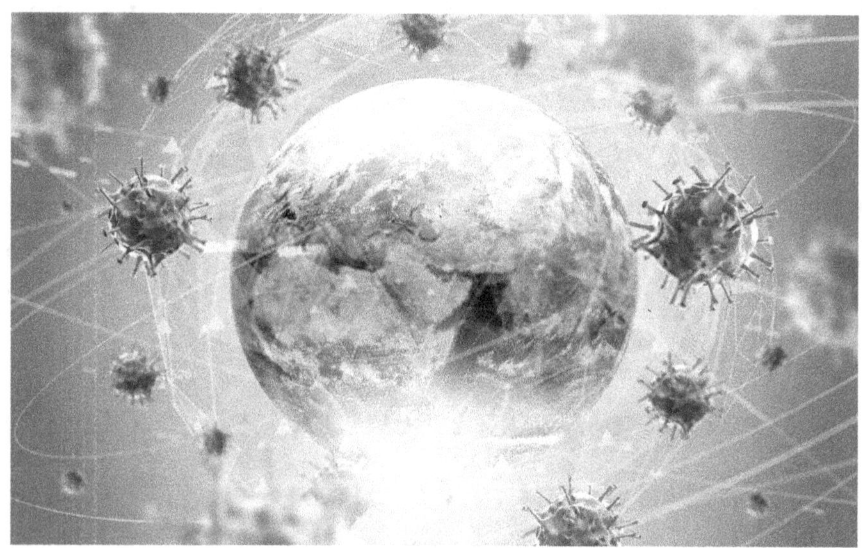

We assumed that coronavirus was a new term, but we can understand that it's a group of viruses when we dig in for details. They are the reasons for deadly diseases caused by birds, animals, and humans. If we look at how humans are infected, it is mainly through the airborne fluid droplets that are from an infected person.

Although there are many types of coronaviruses, we are going to talk about the main seven viruses. Out of these seven viruses, 4 types are seasonal, and they cause flu-like problems. The other three are quite dangerous, and they cause serious issues. There could be deaths if these viruses are left untreated.

The less dangerous viruses are:

- NL63 (alpha coronavirus)
- 229E (alpha coronavirus)
- HKU1 (beta coronavirus)
- OC43 (beta coronavirus)

The dangerous viruses we are talking about are:

- SARS-CoV-2 (covid-19)

- MERS (Middle East respiratory syndrome)

- SARS (severe acute respiratory syndrome)

There have been a lot of deaths caused by these viruses, and most deaths are quite complicated. It is often associated with damaging the systems in our bodies. However, you shouldn't feel demotivated because there several real-life experiences shared how people fought against the virus.

Some of us might wonder why it is termed as coronavirus. There should be some reasons to name it that way. If we look at theories and studies, there is actually a valid reason for the virus to carry the name "coronavirus." The virus got its name in the 1960s because of its crown like structure. Crown is termed as "coronam" in Latin, which is why the virus gets its name. The sugary proteins in the virus are seen through a microscope as spikes. So its structure is the main reason for the virus to get its name. Apart from that, another interesting factor about this virus is it is RNA based.

They are known as genuses, and the four types are:

- Alphacoronavirus (infects mammals and humans)

- Betacoronavirus (infects mammals and humans)

- Gammacoronavirus (infects birds)

- Deltacoronavirus (infects mammals and birds)

The subtypes mentioned above are scientific classification used in order to classify species. As we said, seven viruses impact humans, while three viruses take more percentage on severity. However, these viruses cause mild illness in the airways, throat, lungs, nose, and sinuses. There are instances when these viruses affect the lungs and cause death.

It is clear that coronavirus isn't a new thing

for humans because it has always been there. To be more precise, it has been in the world for more than 50 years. Currently, we all are dealing with COVID-19 that has taken us by surprise. This was first found in Wuhan in 2019 December. Although initial findings were linked to bats, it was then denied because of not having proper evidence concerning it.

The number of positive cases is on the rise, while the mortality rate is varying with time. At the time of writing, there are around 1.52M deaths due to COVID-19. Apart from that, there have been challenges for social activities and economies as well. Although there are vaccines in development, the Pfizer vaccine has been initially sent to the U.K.

This is pretty much about the COVID-19 virus and how it's affecting the world. There are other severe viruses such as SARS and MERS. Let's talk a little bit about them:

- SARS- This was found in Southern China in 2002. Although there have been many studies to track the source of the virus, it still unfounded. The virus turned out a pandemic when there were above 8000 infections in around 26 countries. The infection passed on to humans after infecting animals, and it took about 800 human lives by 2003.

- MERS- The first case of MERS was found in 2012 in Saudi Arabia. Symptoms including cough, fever, diarrhea, and difficulty in breathing were found in infected people. Even with MERS, there were many studies to find the initial case, but evidence suggests that it is related to camels. There were more than 2400 infections in around 27 countries. The pandemic led to 860 deaths.

Now that you know the types of viruses, you can focus on how it gets transmitted to humans. Initially, it was said that the virus was from animals, but no data were supporting the argument. One of the viruses discussed was related to camels, whereas others were assumed to be from cats, bats, and others. No matter what causes the disease, it is important to bear in mind that coronavirus isn't less dangerous than influenza.

Most people assume that coronavirus is better than influenza, but it's not the case. They have different levels of severity. Flu and viruses can create upper respiratory infections while making it contagious. If people associate one another closely, they might contract it, and the symptoms of the virus and flu are quite similar such as tiredness, fever, and cough.

Anyway, there are significant differences between viruses and flu. Especially talking about COVID-19, they can be deadlier than flu, although some conspiracies assume that it is not. The current virus has caused more death than the common flu; therefore, we cannot consider it less risky. Moreover, unlike the common cold, the incubation period for COVID-19 is longer. Thus, the transmission can be unidentified, which is the reason to follow public health measures as said by the authorities.

You might now understand that COVID-19 and flu are dangerous unless adequately treated. But if we pull COVID-19 out of context, it works a bit differently than other viruses. Let's now see how it works on the human body.

How COVID-19 impact the human body?

Although every virus blocks your lungs and airways, let's talk about coronavirus. It definitely does impact your airways and lungs and leads you to fight for breath. One of the most common misconceptions related to COVID-19 is that people assume that everyone will show symptoms upon being infected. But that's not how it works; even if you are infected, there are chances for your body to cover up the symptoms because of your body's immunity levels.

Some people might have caught the virus, but

they wouldn't show any symptoms, and the disease could also be cured without needing hospitalization. This could be because of the mild illness caused by the virus. However, pneumonia is a severe illness caused by COVID-19. Once you get pneumonia, it gets a bit hard to keep your lungs from working as usual because the virus tends to hurt the major parts of your lungs. There are instances when the lungs give up supporting the body with the oxygen required.

Some people might experience the symptoms within 5 days, whereas some might experience it after 12-14 days. While the incubation period is calculated on average, some cases took more than 70 days. However, if people don't show any symptoms, a test could identify if they have contracted the virus.

If you have a great immune system, the virus will take some time to damage your organs, whereas a compromised immune system will easily let in the virus. Once the virus enters your body, it will disturb the air, leading to cough, sore throat, blocked nose, or runny nose. The symptoms may vary from person to person.

When the immune system responds, cytokine production takes place. This production supports cell communication, although lethargy, headaches, fatigue, and muscle aches might be some of the adverse effects of it. Some people might experience diarrhea and nausea if their gut is infected. There are instances when you might experience inflammation due to immune response, and it might even lead to damaged lungs. Thus, a CT scan or X-ray might reveal these damages. COVID-19 pneumonia causes damages to the outer or lower part of your lungs, and these could be identified from a CT scan.

There are hopeless cases when the lungs give up supporting the body, so ventilators support patients in such cases. However, it's important to visit or contact a medical specialist when you or your loved ones experience any symptoms related to COVID-19. Or if a person has come in contact with an infected individual, it's important to do the needful. To be honest, it's always better to be safe than to worry later. Thus, we'll discuss some of the public health measures and personal health measures you must follow.

Public and Person Health Measures

Although scientists have developed relatively effective vaccines, you still need to follow public health measures. Maintaining distance, masking, and following other health measures will not only break the chain. If the vaccines are not as safe as claimed, you can still be on the safe grounds. As said by the CDC, the following are the best ways to stay away from the virus:

Hand washing

- Washing the hands frequently (20 seconds)

- Using alcohol-based sanitizer or soap and water to clean the hands.

- Making sure to wash the hands after going in public, sneezing, coughing, prepping food, eating, using the toilet, interacting with pets, taking care of a sick, and adjusting the face mask.

Maintaining distance

- Staying 2 meters or 6 feet away in public or workplace.

- Avoid physical contact with the sick or, if taking care of the sick, take necessary measures.

- When socializing, maintaining distance while covering the mouth and nose.

Personal health measure

- Disinfect surfaces that get touched frequently, such as doors, phones, door handles, tables, and toilets.

- Use water and soap to clean the surfaces before using a disinfectant.

- Sneeze into your elbow without using the hands, and more importantly, avoid touching the face out of habit.

These are the main health measures that you

need to follow if you want to stay safe. Apart from these, you need to know when to require medical intervention.

If you are experiencing symptoms, you shouldn't visit the doctor. Instead, call him/her and describe your illness so that they will guide you to do the needful. It's important to stay away from other members of your family if you are experiencing the symptoms. Also, don't forget to wear a mask even if you are at home. Some people recover at home without requiring medical treatment. But such people need to follow the health measures accordingly.

However, if you have trouble breathing or if you are experiencing severe chest pain, make sure to call 911 for quick medical intervention. The emergency service providers are aware of the steps to be taken, so you don't have to worry if you have called them.

Chapter 2 – Covid-19 Conspiracy Theories

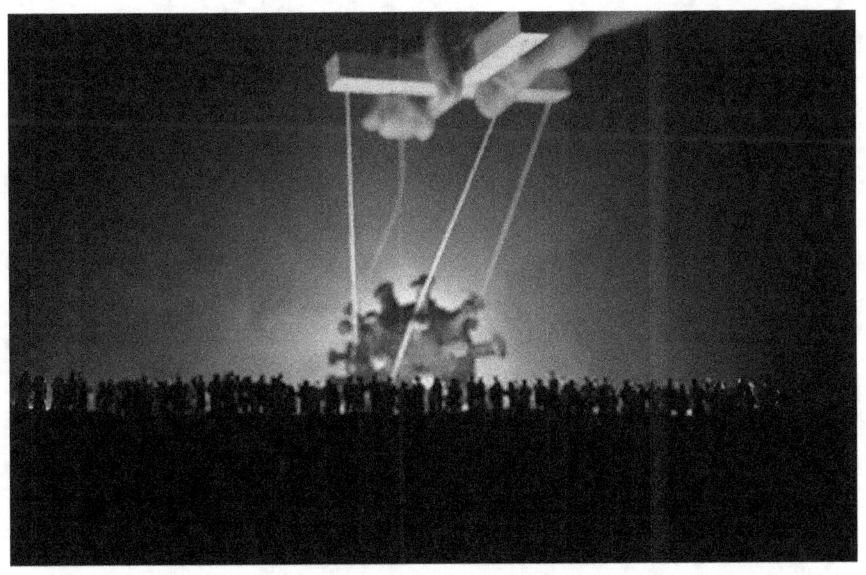

There is a rise in conspiracy theories along with rise in COVID-19 cases. While some might ignore conspiracy theories, most people get affected by them. They find it hard to handle conspiracies.

Do you know what conspiracy theories are? They are basically situations or events manipulated by certain powerful parties with negative intentions. There are six common things in almost all the conspiracy theories and they are:

- Secret plot.

- A team of conspirators.

- Proofs that support their assumption.

- They create false concepts saying that everything is interconnected and no event or situation is an accident.

- They set aside things as good or bad.

- Certain groups and people become the scapegoats.

Conspiracies gain so much recognition because of the way it is portrayed. Most of the time logical explanation of situations and events appear to be true and it gets difficult to prove otherwise. Moreover, it is tough to bring these theories under control as people consume it sooner than true information. At a critical time like COVID-19, it is important to advice people regarding conspiracies because this is a very new thing for everyone.

Conspiracies take root super easily because the parties that trigger any situation or event make sure to do their research. They know the ones who are going to consume their plan so it is easy for them to force in evidence to make it "look" true. Once this is done, conspiracy theories will spread like wildfire.

There are different reasons as to why people spread these theories. Some believe that these are true whereas some try to provoke or manipulate a target audience. There could be financial or political reasons for spreading these theories. Thus, you have to be careful when you are subjected to believe conspiracies. However, UNESCO and the European Commission have published educational infographics that will help you understand and debunk conspiracy theories.

Now, let's check some of the common conspiracy theories related to COVID-19.

Accidental virus leak in Wuhan

It is no wonder that the conspiracy theory of virus being leaked in Wuhan started taking turns in the world. The Trump administration has always been fueled up with conspiracies and the same administration has triggered this conspiracy theory through racist remark such as "Wuhan virus," "China Virus" or "Kung Flu." While the administration had no proofs to back up their claim, it still kept circulating.

The Wuhan Institute of Virology (WIV) scientists refuted the claim over and over stating that it is merely a conspiracy theory. During the meeting conducted by NBC News channel, the vice director of the institute, Yuan Zhiming denied the claim repeatedly while stating that the first sample was obtained only after the first case was reported in Wuhan.

He also added, "I have repeatedly emphasized that it was on December 30 that we got contact with the samples of SARS-like pneumonia or pneumonia of unknown cause sent from the hospital. We have not encountered the novel coronavirus before that, and without this virus, there is no way that it is leaked from the lab."

Along with that, President of EcoHealth Alliance, Peter Daszak who worked with the institute for more than 16 years rejected the claim made concerning the virus leak from the lab. He mentioned that, "The fact that they published the sequence so quickly suggests to me that they weren't trying to cover up anything," he further added, "absolutely zero evidence that it escaped from a lab."

All in all, the director of U.S. National Institute of Allergy and Infectious Diseases, Anthony Fauci, said that there are no evidence that the virus leaked from the lab.

Secret Bio Weapon of Mass Destruction

Another common conspiracy theory is that COVID-19 is a secret bio weapon for mass destruction. It is said that the bio weapon was intentionally introduced by the Chinese scientists. As per the study done by Pew Research, three out of ten Americans believe the conspiracy theory that the virus was created in a lab. Further, 23% of believe that the virus was created on purpose and 6% of them believe that it's an accident.

This conspiracy theory was somehow made popular by the US politics. The mainstream light was on the news because of US Sen. Tom Cotton who emphasized the theories in one of the conservative media outlets, Washington Examiner that WIV is connected to Beijing's bio weapon program.

However, by now, there are a lot of theories

to debunk the claim made because there are no evidence that this was produced as a bio weapon.

End of the World

A higher percentage of people is anticipating that this is going to be the end of the world. COVID-19 is considered one of the signs that the end is nearing. Some conspiracy theorists say that end times are nearing and it is written in the bible. They have come into realization that the outbreak is prewritten and it is bound to happen.

End Times Truth, a Christian website says, "The prophets saw a time of tremendous upheaval and destruction just before the end of this age."

They also added, "Jesus predicted that immediately before He returns the world would experience a time of trouble unparalleled in history where all life would be threatened."

The website discussed about the world war that might be triggered very soon. To be precise, it was termed as, "In the Bible, this time is called the Great Tribulation. The prophets predicted that it would start with a war in the Middle East and lead to a global battle."

However, none of these have been backed up by proof.

5G causes COVID-19

The very reason for this conspiracy theory is that many cities in China have rolled out 5G before the outbreak in Wuhan. Another take on this theory is that 5G weakens the human's immune system. Hence, they become vulnerable to the virus.

This is conspiracy theory is outright falls because there is evidence to prove that 5G could damage your immune system. Electromagnetic spectrum consists of non-ionizing and ionizing radiation. We all know that ionizing radiation is riskier with increased frequencies such as UVB and UVA rays. So this can damage the DNA and constant damages to the DNA might lead to cancer. This is why frequent X-rays is not healthy.

Contrastingly, the 5G technology has non-ionizing radiations with less frequencies so it doesn't have the capacity to damage human DNA. People carry the similar fear for phone radiation but it has now been discredited because there is no proper data to prove the claim that radiation can cause tissue damage.

However, there are no quality studies to find whether the mobile phones are unsafe as they claim. There are no cases related to cancers or brain tumors because of prolonged phone usage. Thus, the takeaway is that even if there are risks in using mobile phones that would be relatively lower and weak.

Moreover, there is no link between COVID-19 and 5G network. If we are to worry about something, it could be the environmental crisis and air pollution, it has more scientific backups.

Cleaning up the "Golden Billion"

This is an interesting concept to learn about because this is not the first time that the "Golden Billion" is surfacing the internet. It has been resurfacing time to time when tough time is ahead. This is considered as an alleged project run by the rich to reduce the population so that the privileged inhabitants will prevail on Earth. The phrase "Golden Billion" was found in the book "The Conspiracy of the World Government" which was written by Anatoly Kuzmich Tsikonov.

The very reason that the "Golden Billion" is making rounds is because of the coronavirus. Conspiracy is that this is a strategy for global scale depopulation. It's pretty easy to understand why conspirators assume it that way.

They claim that the virus is produced on purpose although evidence say otherwise. According to them, this is a biological weapon but scientists have disagreed and proved that it is not. As the virus would kill older generation, it is possible to save pension funds so that's a positive impact for the economy. But this is not certainly true because the risk is high on young adults too. They believe that the rich can protect themselves with premium healthcare, isolation, home quarantine, and so on. But based on the researches, the virus transmits to people regardless of their wealth, age, sex, and social status.

Bill Gates is Responsible for the Virus

Along with David Icke, many other people

accused Gates. They claimed that he is responsible for the virus. According to their claim, Bill Gates's plot was to produce vaccines and insert microchips in humans so that he can control the world. Apart from conspiracy theorists, religious leaders too linked it to Biblical prophecy. Most Americans rejected the need for masks, lockdowns, and vaccines, even if they get approved vaccines.

Not only Americans, but many other parts of the world were also against public health measures, which led to many issues, including a spike in positive cases. Political leaders further fueled the conspiracy theory. They motivated people to try medicines that weren't approved by the FDA and other traditional medicines.

COVID-19 is less harmful than seasonal flu

Since the start of COVID-19, this conspiracy theory is on the top, and it doesn't look like people will stop spreading it. If you think logically, you would understand that this is a clear cut falsehood because we've lost so many lives to COVID-19, including frontline workers. One of the tweets that triggered the conspiracy was Donald Trump's, and it is was, "So last year 37,000 Americans died from the common flu. It averages between 27,000 and 70,000 per year. Nothing is shut down, life & the economy go on. At this moment, there are 546 confirmed cases of Coronavirus, with 22 deaths. Think about that!"

However, the numbers mentioned were CDC's algorithm on CDC's influenza burden, so they are not considered real deaths. It's the stats based on speculations of unreported cases. The CDC reported the flu and pneumonia death count in Michigan from the 1st of February, 2020 to the 25th of April, 2020, there were 220 flu deaths and 2559 pneumonia, and 834 deaths had COVID-19 and pneumonia. Although the statics are based on Michigan's death count, almost all the states have more COVID-19 deaths than season flu deaths. Hence, it's false that COVID-19 is less risky than seasonal flu.

On Forbes, the post about The Most Common Coronavirus Conspiracies Circulating In The Media [Infographic] offers more insights into this, so try taking a look at it.

"Conspiracy theories cause real harm to people, to their health, and also to their physical safety. They amplify and legitimize misconceptions about the pandemic, and reinforce stereotypes which can fuel violence and violent extremist ideologies." –**UNESCO Director-General**

Chapter 3 – The Future After COVID-19

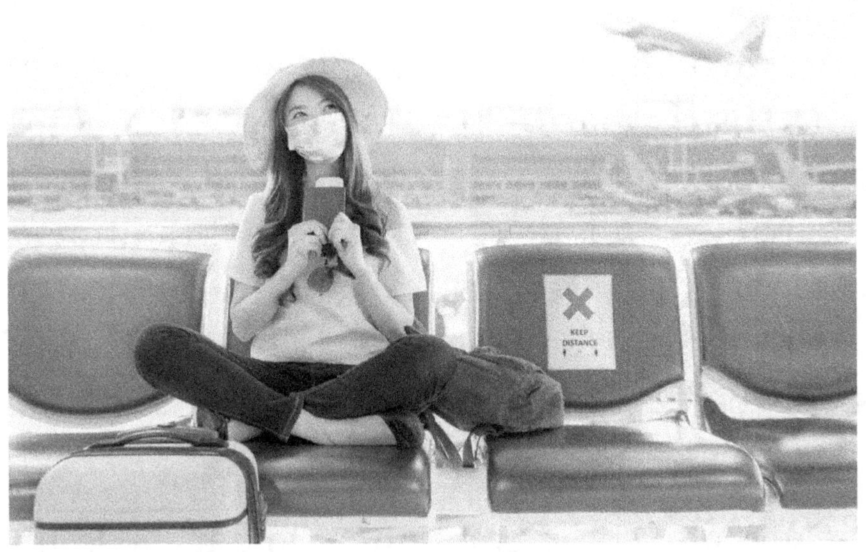

We talk about the pandemic, but we also think about how lives would be after COVID-19. Just like for everything else in life, COVID-19, too, will have an after phase. What are your thoughts on how the future after the pandemic would be? Although we are adapting to the 'new normal,' we are still in the denial stage. It will take some time to accept the new living style, but we'll get there over time because we have to.

One of the things that we cannot get rid of any time soon is masks. Even if the vaccines become successful, we might still have to wear the mask until the public authorities say otherwise. Apart from masking, we might have to adapt to a new working style. Some companies might go back to traditional working style, yet they'd have to follow the health measures. This might lead to a lot of inconveniences while creating more costs for the organization.

Meanwhile, some companies might focus on a hybrid remote-office style. This is an excellent method to control costs while keeping the workflow like it used to be. When companies adopt this style, they'll be able to set aside days to meet as a team, which is an essential factor.

However, when we look at social media accounts, it's clear that people are missing their regular working style. Although they've complained about how going to the office has been hectic, now they worry about missing it. Office goers are looking forward to engaging with teammates physically because virtual meetings have become melancholic. However, when we consider the number of cases worldwide, it doesn't look as if the work culture would come back to normal.

Since the pandemic was announced, there have been a lot of ups and downs. Some people lost their jobs while some improved themselves to secure better jobs. Many businesses came up with new ideas, while others had nothing else to do than keep their businesses halted. Likewise, there have been a lot of changes in lifestyles. Some people enjoyed the change, and some enjoyed the break unasked for. Simultaneously, some had a hard time managing lives with their savings. All in all, working from home became a thing that 90% of the businesses followed. Right now, most companies are following the WFH system because there are no other better options.

When we think of the post-pandemic situation, it might need heavy changes in the system. Even if companies decide to go back to a typical working style, there would be many changes. They might have to bear a cost when following public health measures. If required, they might have to bear the cost of immediate PCR testing and self-quarantine procedures, and so on.

The HR department will have a lot of changes when planning, managing and recruiting. The future of work will not be the same because the pandemic has created the need for a change. When the businesses plan for the post-COVID-19 situation, they need to inform the employees in due course. When the employees understand the change, they will realize the ways to fit in. Along with all the other changes, the companies are more interested in contingent workers than full-time workers because it saves them a lot of money.

Brain Kopp, who is the Vice President of Gartner, mentions, "HR leaders who respond effectively can ensure their organizations stand out from competitors." It's understandable why HR leaders have to play a major role during this pandemic. If the companies want to stand out, they must be ready to become the one-of-a-kind service provider.

It's evident that work will never look like it was. There will be differences even if you don't want to accept the changes. If the organizations understand that the work will never be the same, they will focus on restructuring the organization. Many well-established business people say that the change is undeniable. We cannot disagree that the change has caused many inconveniences in people's lives, but on a positive note, new ideas can be tried and tested during this time.

As the long adapted 9-5 work style has been halted, it's time for the organizations to check whether their new ideas might work. Or they can test whether the WFH concept could work in the long run. According to the current stats, it's said that the WFH concept has increased work efficiency in many employees. It has also become a factor to support the self-development of the employees. They have no other choice than to take responsibility for the work assigned while handling the household chores. The best thing about the WFH concept is that it has highlighted that the bureaucracy isn't essential. If a leader has proactive thoughts, he will realize that this is not the time to worry about the change; rather, this is the time to plan on overcoming the hurdle.

How Can Employers Manage Post COVID-19 Workspace?

As we discussed, change is undeniable, so we have to prepare ourselves to face it. Different companies have different plans concerning their workplace. Some might keep their business closed until a 100% effective vaccine has been found and might adapt to WFH. Or they might even consider it a better option than working in physical offices or companies.

Meanwhile, some might reopen their businesses by taking necessary health measures even though it can increase the company's cost. Regardless of your business's category, you have to take the measures needed to ensure that employees have a safe workspace. We'll discuss some of the measures that employers can take to manage the workspace.

- Involve your team in decision making-

We often see leaders who hardly involve their team in decision making. But COVID-19 has taught us the right way to make a decision. The pandemic has made us work as a team, and companies realize its importance now more than ever. Teamwork has always been an integral part of success. But during this pandemic, many companies faced tough times because they couldn't bring the team together to perform as one unit.

This should be a lesson when carrying forward your business after the pandemic. While it's important to work as a team, it is also important to create rules for the post-pandemic workspace. When you open your business after the pandemic, you need to gather your team. Talk about the rules that you already had. Discuss with your team the new rules that you are planning to impose. Make sure that the team members are in a position to abide by the rules.

If you plan to carry on the hybrid remote-office work, you must ensure that the respective team leaders have discussed the meetings and other essential details with their team. The post-pandemic work environment will have many differences; therefore, it's vigilant to discuss everything before working.

- Treat employee's wellbeing as a top priority

If there's one thing the whole world understood, it could be that wellbeing is our most treasured wealth. Even businesses started realizing how important it is to give priority to one's health. Although it became a concern before COVID-19, after the COVID-19 situation, employers will spend more interest on employee wellbeing.

For example, Deloitte believes that prioritizing employees' wellbeing directly impact their organization's success. If we think about how organizations were performing before COVID-19, employees' wellbeing was limited to paid or non-paid sick leave. But now, the need to focus on wellbeing has moved from papers to hearts. This means every team leader must make an effort to connect with the team to understand how they are doing.

This is not going to be easy, but it's worth the effort because mental health is crucial. If you want your team members to perform well, you need to do what it takes. We understand that the pandemic has taken a toll on everyone's mental health. If you are planning to reopen after the pandemic, you need to know that employees have had a hard time during the pandemic. Their mental health has been jeopardized because of a sudden change in the work style.

Hence, you need to take measures to avoid it when you begin working after the pandemic. Though it might be an additional duty to a leader's role, it's unavoidable. Some leaders maintain a checklist to make sure that they are keeping up with the team members. If a team member is not performing as he is used to performing, it's important to have a one-on-one conversion to identify the underlying problem. So if you want to run your business after the pandemic successfully, you need to hone these skills.

- Let the team members feel their belongingness

Some organizations would have respected and valued employees even before the pandemic, but most organizations fail to do it. One of the reasons employees don't give their best is that they don't feel like they belong to the team. They don't feel appreciated or respected by the team members and the leaders.

The pandemic has made us realize that belongingness is vital. During the pandemic, every team member had to work from home, which would have pushed them to loneliness. It made us understand why we need to make every team member feel that they are essential and their work is appreciated.

When the team members feel they belong to the group, they tend to put their hearts and souls into the work. This eventually increases the efficiency. Therefore, when you reopen after the pandemic, make sure to value the employees working for the organization.

- Train employees to adapt to the ongoing changes

The pandemic is a lesson that nothing stays the same. We cannot expect the work culture to be the same. When we look at the changes that have already happened, it is clear that there will be many more changes. Employees need to adapt to these changes if they want to secure their jobs, and it's in the hands of employers to train them.

The business world is experiencing a digital transformation, and slowly but steadily, Artificial Intelligence will come into play. Although it was assumed that the AI would replace employees, luckily, it seems as if it's not going to happen. Instead of replacing, AI will augment workers to perform better.

As digital transformation is apparent, team leaders or employers must do the needful to train the employees to adapt to it. They need to find out the areas that the team members are good at and hone their skills through different training sessions. This is the best time to help your employees' upskill, and this will eventually become beneficial to your organization.

As you would have anticipated, the business world is rapidly changing. If you are not ready to pace along, it will be impossible to continue your journey. Moreover, it's wiser to be prepared than to regret it later. This is the best time to experiment and implement, so do it wisely. Make sure to create a workspace that your employees feel safe and productive. While you create a safe workspace for your employees, make sure to take a look at CDC's Interim Guidance for Businesses and Employers Responding to Coronavirus Disease 2019 (COVID-19), May 2020.

How Can Employees Manage Post COVID-19 Workspace?

We've learned employer's take on post-pandemic workspace. Now, let's talk about employees and how they must prepare themselves to manage post-pandemic workspace. COVID-19 has taught us that technology skills are essential, and having a plan B is crucial in a rapidly changing world.

While certain parts of the world have overcome the pandemic up to some extent, some countries are still struggling with the pandemic. However, when talking about how employees must prepare themselves for the post-pandemic workspace, the following factors are considered more important:

- Sharpening the technological skills

Although we wouldn't have considered technological skills before COVID-19, it has now become important. Even if the companies decide to reopen, certain tools like a project management tool, time tracking tool, etc., might not go out of the picture. Likewise, there are certain types of software that are adopted by companies, so it makes things tough for employees without technological skills. This is the main reason to improve your technological skills. Even though it sounds unfair to employees in rural areas, there are no better options. The world is digitizing, so we have to upgrade ourselves to fit in.

- Hone your communication skill

It's hard to persist in the business world if you don't have excellent communication skills. But it will become harder after the pandemic. Currently, WFH has become the main working style, so if you cannot communicate with your team, it will become challenging to complete a task. You might say that communication skill is anyway, important. Of course, it is. You need to have the skill even before the pandemic, but working in a physical office and communicating with your manager might not be the same in a virtual working environment. Hence, you need to fine-tune your communication skill by analyzing the hurdles you face in a virtual working environment.

- Have a plan B even if you have a day job

We do not suggest doing freelancing if you don't want to, but you must have a plan B. Many people have lost their jobs during the pandemic, and many have faced a financial crisis. If you don't want to struggle without money, you need to have a backup plan. While you work on your day job, try to find other ways to increase your income, such as passive income. Pandemic is a reminder and a lesson that we must be prepared for.

These skills will help us understand the ways to fight the changes that impact the world. Once you master the skills, you will no longer shy away from making decisions when situations like COVID-19 take place; instead, you will thrive.

Next, let's learn about the education of the future.

Chapter 4 – Education of the Future – How Education will Change After COVID-19

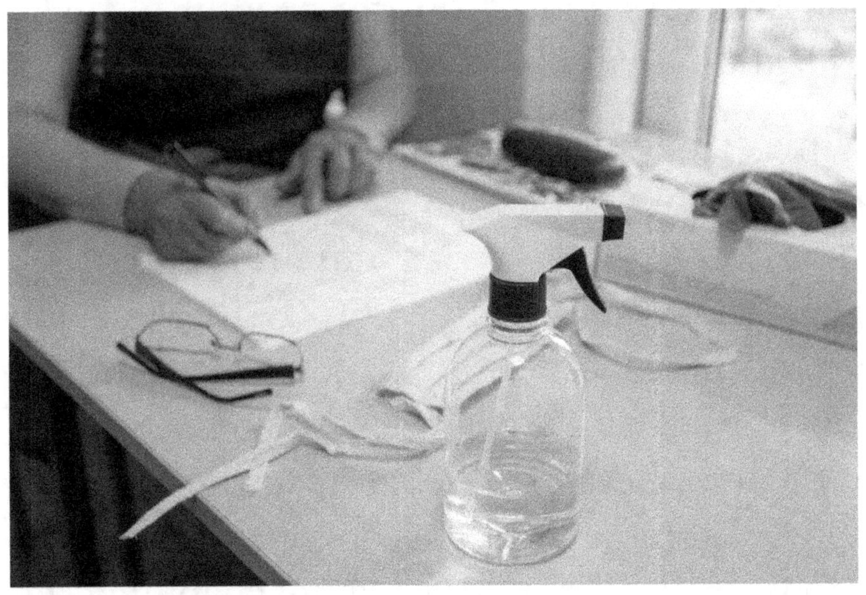

Next to working, education has changed drastically because of the pandemic. Students and educators worldwide are facing a massive shift in the typical educational style. While the schools remained closed, teaching has been shifted to digital platforms. Though teaching online isn't a viable solution, there are no better options to keep the education industry moving. Online education isn't for everyone because not every student can afford it; this is why we need to build back better, at least after COVID-19. The policymakers should do the needful to make education accessible to every student.

While some countries have reopened the school, some others have kept schools closed for safety. However, it's important to think about the situation after COVID-19. How will education be after the pandemic? Can you expect a lot of changes? There could be a lot of changes because it's better to be safe than sorry. Therefore, schools might follow strict public health measures while changing the education system to match the changed lifestyle.

Many studies are carried on to find the best ways to educate students while ensuring their safety. These studies try to find solutions that will work even if the world is bombarded with another crisis. They want to make sure that the students get to educate themselves regardless of the situation. There are a lot of insights on this topic that I can share with you, but some of the prominent ones are as below:

Digitalizing will become a priority

Thinking about the future of education is crucial because it definitely needs a transformation. Now that the world has become more digitalized and COVID-19 has proved it further, now is the best time to use the technology in the education industry. Students should get access to the upgraded learning system because now education is more than writing, reading, and arithmetic. It should have another element –rethinking.

Using technology to empower rethinking is a vigilant choice, and it should be done in a way that doesn't create adverse effects. However, using technology to educate students will offer choices; they can either choose remote learning or in-class learning. It's better to prioritize students' comfort levels so that there will be an increase in the output.

Currently, online learning has become the only choice in most countries, but it will become one of the choices available for students over time. It will offer the feasibility of holding video conferences, assessment tools, and feedback tools.

Even if the pandemic ends, it's better to prioritize safety, so holding meetings online could be a good choice. Already there are several studies underway to ensure that digitizing will work for students and educators equally. It is also important to know that some traditional teaching methodologies might still work even after the pandemic.

- A drastic change in the academic calendar

Schools are struggling to meet a term's work and tick off dates in the academic calendar because of COVID-19. It has become a massive challenge to educate students while ensuring that they have learned and understood what's being taught. Doing Zoom classes have been a chore for most teachers who are not comfortable with the technology, but some tips and tricks will make Zoom sessions easier.

However, we cannot say that the Zoom classes will end with the pandemic because there are chances that it might remain even after the pandemic. Schools may start earlier than usual and try to complete a term's work in a short time. The holidays will be changed by considering the seasons that link to seasonal flu.

There will be changes in the number of students per classroom, overcrowded classrooms will be split into two or more, and there will be social distancing. Students will be advised to follow safety measures regardless of the situation.

- Classrooms will become open and collaborative

Although classrooms already have open and collaborative discussions, it wasn't effectively followed. But one of the anticipations is that after COVID-19, the classrooms will become more collaborative and open.

Students must be taught question what they learn and should have the knowledge to filter authentic and reliable information. Also, teachers should motivate and encourage students to stay connected to the digital world healthily. Since the world values teamwork, teachers should improve collaboration and teamwork in future education.

- Health over everything else

Students and teachers' health will be prioritized over everything else because why not? COVID-19 has taught us that heath is more important than anything else. It might become a rule to do COVID-19 testing in the school.

Meanwhile, social distancing, masking, and regular hand washing are some of the rules that must be followed unless the WHO says otherwise. Classrooms will be shifted into more open spaces. Hence, it's easy to promote interactive learning.

These are some of the changes that we are most likely to witness in the education of the future. There is an interesting article on the UNESCO blog that you might like reading – Build back better: Education must change after COVID-19 to meet the climate crisis.

Conclusion

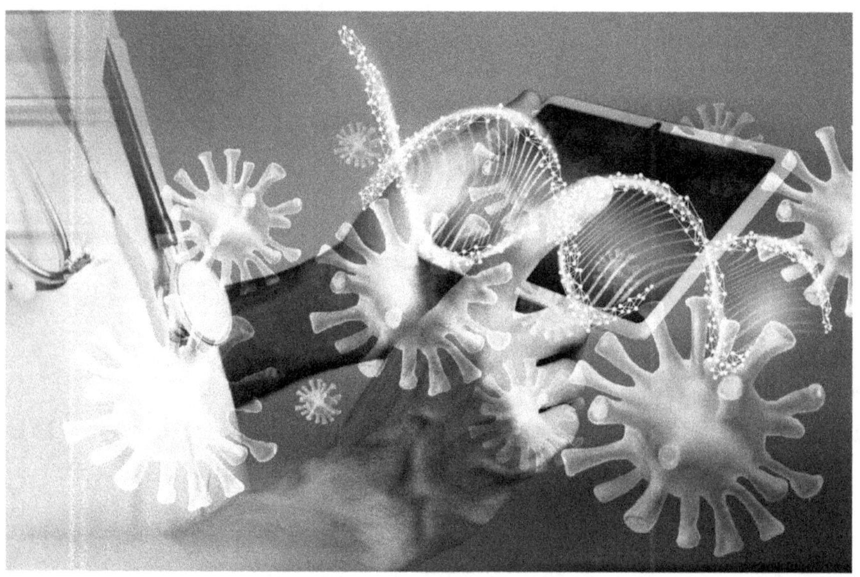

The world lost around 1 million people, and most COVID-19 deaths were too painful to hear without getting teary-eyed. If you read this article titled "3,000 people have died from COVID-19 in Wisconsin. Here are stories of 6 lives lost," I'm sure you'll understand the depth of the virus better than you did before. Or, if you have denied it so far, these real-life experiences will prove your understanding wrong.

However, there's another side to the virus; it's not as if everyone who gets the virus dies. Of course, there are survivors and recoveries. More than 38.3M people have recovered from the virus, which is more than the rate of deaths. But you shouldn't be carefree as there are more recoveries than death because some COVID-19 survivors say that they touched death. This certainly means that the struggle was real, and they had a hard time fighting the virus.

The piece on "A coronavirus survivor's story: 'I touched death'" would give you chills and tears when you continue reading it. However, I urge people to read because it makes you realize that you need to have faith and hope to fight the virus.

It is essential to understand the depth of the virus while educating yourself on the misinformation. This short eBook includes all the information from conspiracies to misinformation so that you can find everything in one place.

I hope this eBook provides information that will clear your doubts and offer credible information.

I hope, that you really enjoyed reading my book.

Thanks for buying the book anyway!